The

Psychology

of

Top Talent

The Practical Scientifically Proven Method to Identify,
Hire, and Develop High Performers

DR. ERIC FRAZER

CONTENTS

BULK PURCHASES & SPEAKING

For information about discounts for bulk purchases, or to invite

Dr. Frazer to speak at your company,

e-mail speaking@hiringtoptalent.com or call 203-400-6204.

FOREWORD-SEIZE YOUR MOMENT

In the 2018 Disney-Pixar movie *Coco,* a prevailing theme of the story is personified by one of the main characters, Ernesto de la Cruz, who emulates the saying, "Seize Your Moment," as a mantra for his own success and the inspiration for others. It captures the dream of twelve-year-old Miguel. In the story, Miguel believes this man is his great-great-grandfather, a famous musician, but Miguel later learns of another backstory. Hector, a man portrayed in the film as being forgotten, was Ernesto's former partner musician. Ernesto murdered Hector so he could keep all of the fame and fortune to himself. Hector, not Ernesto, was actually Miguel's great-great-grandfather.

There are many layers to this psychological cake. Quite simply we can all take away the notion of wanting to seize our own moments, though the warning in the movie also holds true—not at the expense of greed nor, of course, murder. In modern day, this type of murder comes from slander, deceit, conning, and anything else that would be considered unethical business.

To truly seize our moment, the movie reminds us we must identify our gift, which in this story is musicianship. From there, to be truly great, we must practice. I will break down this technique and demonstrate how psychological research has proven practice to be a timeless secret for the most successful people. In this book, I will leverage the aggregate of research on top talent and weave it together into meaningful, applicable points for you to examine in your own life reflectively, followed by practical skills, exercises, habits, and organizational strategies to fully optimize yourself as an individual, a professional, and an organizational leader.

You can use this book in any way you wish, but to reap its full benefits, the approach I recommend is akin to the one I outline throughout it—break down your actions into bite-size achievable steps, which serve as your practice at self-mastery, discipline, and performance enhancement.

With so many personal and professional technology distractions simultaneously testing your self-control and attention all day, focus is even more difficult to achieve than ever. I will show you how to develop this level of focus in yourself, identify it in others, and cultivate it in your organization.

Set your first goal to finish this book by a certain date. This book has ten chapters, and by immediately scheduling ten reading sessions at your own pace, you can easily accomplish this goal and be on your way toward learning and implementing the changes to seize your moment.

CHAPTER 1

THE PSYCHOLOGICAL PROFILE OF TOP TALENT

The Personal Self

The Personal Self is who we are, and to develop the Professional Self and Organization Self, it is imperative to work on all three in harmony. You cannot expect to "get ahead" by simply working to close deals and complete projects. You, in the broadest sense, are a manifestation of everything you bring to the table— namely your character.

How does one develop character? We are all made up of various personality facets: character strengths and liabilities. We engage in the development of the Personal Self by enhancing our strengths and appreciating (a term I will come back to later) our liabilities. We sand down our liabilities with deliberate practice (another term I will come back to later) so they are smooth like glass and create minimal, if any, resistance for ourselves and others.

I drink my own Kool-Aid, and yes, my own psychotherapy has proven highly beneficial as one mechanism to varnish personal liabilities. Many others agree with the notion that psychotherapy is an invaluable tool for personal development. One example is Debbie Millman.

For its price, psychotherapy is a bargain. Given the prevalence of mental illness and addiction in our society, combined with the abrasive personality features we all possess to some extent, there is only gain to be had. I was once coaching a technology executive who was secretly suffering from episodes of depression in spite of a career and family life that would have been envied by practically anyone. In confidence, we determined he needed a brief course of psychotherapy to treat his depression (without medication, per his preference), which proved to be an efficacious tool. Not only did he participate in the course of treatment, but his career continued to explode and he was tracked into a leadership program, a hefty raise, and promotion to boot.

You may consider yourself well-adjusted. That type of narcissistic thinking falls on the right side of the continuum. You cannot see what you do not see. Narcissism is only one example. Many other personality traits, which you can think of as facets falling on a continuum, may be misaligned in your life. How conscientious are you? Could you do better? Did you fail to connect with someone because of falling short in this area? Did your biases get in the way of being identified for a greater opportunity in your respective professional role? Perhaps you need to do work to be more open- minded. We all possess these kinds of blind spots, to a greater or lesser degree, that first need revelation through discovery in coaching or psychotherapy, followed by action to actually make the change and put these character traits in better harmony.

For a final note on the psychotherapy endeavor, I see many people having just as much misfortune with psychotherapy as they do with any other professional engagement. Often the root of the problem is finding the right match. There are numerous types of evidenced-based therapy—some short term, some long term— which greatly optimize the likelihood of a successful outcome. For example, anxiety and panic is best treated with Cognitive Behavioral Therapy (CBT) or Mindfulness Based Therapy. Similarly, addiction is best treated by an expert in that domain. Check the credentials and expertise of the psychotherapist you choose versus simply relying on the person your best friend has seen. What was good for them is not necessarily good for you.

Another aspect of self-development pertains to the mind. This is a bit of a combination of neuroscience and Buddhist thinking about the concept of mind, but it has been scientifically demonstrated that our minds influence our cells. This can all be simply summed up to mean that you are not your thoughts or feelings. The task is to actually be able to observe your thoughts and feelings in a detached nonjudgmental way. In other words, realize you can have control over both—first by observation and second by non-impulsive action.

For most, this is a lifelong endeavor, but the most important aspect is to simply take action now and start the practice. When you arrive at work and you're feeling tense or having any negative thoughts, the first step is to recognize that neither will get you into the right "state" of mind or body to perform your best. To disengage, as Thich Nhat Hanh teaches in his book *The Miracle of Mindfulness* you can simply breathe. Taking seven slow breaths allows you to put your mind and body back in balance, a kind of reboot. This enables you to observe your thoughts and feelings and puts you in a better physiological state to make an agile and precise shift.

You accomplish two things. First, you relax your body. Second, you relax your mind and give yourself the perspective to change your mind so you may in fact regroup with optimism to create whatever solution you are seeking in that moment. This, of course, can be repeated and practiced regularly. Those wishing to go deeper can engage in routine deep breathing or meditation. The style does not matter. You can use a simple non-secular breathing meditation, in which you simply close your eyes, sit or lie down, and engage in relaxed breathing for five minutes. Those wishing for more of a spiritual twist will find endless opportunities.

In our modern day, we can leverage technology to make this exercise as easy as anything else in our lives. The App Insight Timer can be utilized for any duration of meditation at any time, in silence, with music, with teachings, and the list goes on. I routinely meditate for a minimum of ten minutes first thing in the morning, though it can be done any time your schedule allows. I have also found that having a journal available for meditation is equally useful, as meditation tends to elicit insights, solutions for problems, and other unexpected benefits you will wish to write down for either further reflection or immediate action.

If you don't like the word meditation, you can replace it with mindfulness. From a practical standpoint, they are synonymous. Mindfulness simply means being aware and being present. Being aware and being present means your mind is not distracted, or if it is (which is perfectly normal), you are aware that your mind is distracted. Having that awareness is exactly the enhanced state you are seeking, so you are able to observe and not simply react. This is learning focus. Even doing so for a few minutes gives you perspective and a better capacity for self-discipline and insightful action versus reactive impulsivity.

The third aspect of the Personal Self is physical well-being. High performance requires keeping a steady flow of energy throughout the day, with the goal of eliminating spikes and crashes. Habits like having six Starbucks through mid-day followed by another half-case of Red Bull are foolhardy. Whereas there are endless books—and I will provide a few references for nutrition, endurance training, and the like—the formula for maintaining optimal well-being, like anything else, is proportion. First is sleep, and recognizing your own sleep hygiene needs. Some people need more, other less. The key is not to fight it. Keep a set regimen with minor deviations and of course rule-breaking during vacations and weekends to replenish your needs. Arianna Huffington wrote an entire book on Sleep, *The Sleep Revolution* following what I will refer to as her self- described prolonged redlining followed by a severe physical decline.

Nutrition comes second. The simplest points on this include the following. Drink no less than one liter of water daily. Two is best. You can hold yourself accountable to this by bringing a water bottle with you each day. Consume minimal, if any, refined sugars and particularly no sugar beverages. Coffee can be supplemented with Japanese green tea during the day. Nuts, particularly raw almonds and cashews, make for great snacks during the day, as do natural fruits (apples, oranges, bananas, grapefruit) which are naturally filling and energy producing. Lunches should be revitalizing salads with plenty of raw vegetables, olives, and some sprinkled cheese (I like goat cheese) for flavoring and a minimal amount of dressing.

Evening dinner is an opportunity to expand the palate, but again with attention on eating healthy.

Last, but not least, is exercise. Exercise is proven to raise dopamine, which produces feelings of optimism. I like to exercise in the morning, but that is just my body-rhythm preference. It doesn't matter when it is done as long as it's done. Some interesting studies have shown the effects of very brief exercises having better efficacy than the long, slow cardio workouts of yesteryears. Tim Ferris Show w/ Dr. Martin Gibala.

High performers are always short on time, and this is a great way to squeeze in highly productive workouts even when time is thin. Another opportunity during a day with no opportunity to get outside or get to a gym is to incorporate strength training exercises that will not result in building up a sweat and can be done in about fifteen to twenty minutes. An amazing workout for building your core is freely published here:

https://www.outsideonline.com/1987466/definitive-10-step-guide-building-do-anything-core

There are fair number of so-called cognitive enhancers (nootropics) and related products on the market. High performers are always looking for a "hack" to get a competitive advantage, and this is one of them. I have experimented with many of them, some referred by nutritionists and others that are more mainstream (like lion's mane mushroom), none of which have ever provided me any noticeable benefit. One, in fact, actually made me sleepy! While there is some research on these products, it is very scant. In general, my conclusions for these experiments is that if you are fundamentally a healthy person, and following good physical wellness practices, you are unlikely to receive any noticeable sustained benefit. Nonetheless, everyone is different, so feel free to give one a try and keep an eye on this ever-growing market.

Below is a sample routine that has worked for me. You can establish a similar routine that matches your preferences so you feel good about it.

My Sample Daily High-Performance Routine

10:00 p.m. – 4:45 a.m.: Sleep

4:55 a.m. – 5:35 a.m.: Exercise [Run/Bike/TRX Strength Training]

5:45 a.m. – 6:00 a.m.: Meditation/Journaling

Breakfast: Steel cut oatmeal with fruit, two tablespoons of cinnamon and honey, coffee

Morning Snack: Raw almonds, double espresso

Lunch: Kale with avocado and red peppers, goat cheese, fig balsamic dressing

Afternoon Snack: Apple, brown rice and quinoa packet

Dinner: As preferred

Opt-Ins for Random Benefit and Experimentation

Mid-Day / End of Day Yoga or Mid-Day Meditation Supplements (Vitamin D, Multivitamin + Omega 3s, MSM)

Consult with a local nutritionist Kombucha

Chamomile tea before bed

The Professional Self

Your Professional Self is an extension of your Personal Self. By building off this solid foundation, high performers are well equipped to apply related principles to the workplace. One personality trait that is frequently referred to with a negative connotation is narcissism. However, personality facets need to be understood as dimensional, not categorical. Ironically, one professional group who was shown to have high narcissism on a famous personality test was pilots. Would you want someone who lacks confidence at the stick? The same rationale can be considered for individuals that are being onboarded into leadership roles.

Other distinct personality traits and their accompanying behaviors will be discussed throughout this book, but the point is that finding people with elevated confidence (healthy narcissism) is necessary for ongoing professional development. This type of narcissism is an underpinning for developing expertise—something top talent is known for possessing. Psychologists Angela Duckworth and Barry Kaufman offer one formula for understanding expertise is as follows: Expertise = Talent + Effort.[1]

Finding top talent is challenging enough, but what guarantee do you have that they will demonstrate commensurate effort to develop highly specialized skills? The answer is in past effort. By looking at both personal and professional endeavors in the past, one can appraise how much effort they have put into accomplishing prior goals in tandem with their intrinsic talent. When looking at past accomplishments to gauge how effort was applied and successfully executed, there are three maxims to consider:

1. What evidence is there that they did the work?
2. How did they schedule the work flow to meet deadlines and objectives?
3. How did they tolerate the discomforts from obstacles and solve conflicts that emerged?

The answers to these questions will help you determine whether you not only have a talented candidate, but also one who, whether they know it or not, has a methodology for applying effort to get things

---

[1] https://onlinelibrary.wiley.com/doi/abs/10.1002/wcs.1365 https://scottbarrykaufman.com/wp-content/uploads/2015/09/10.1002_wcs.1365.pdf

done. A former mentor of mine had a very strong opinion about how to deal with competitors. His words were, "Steal them." Not quite literally, but what he meant was "take action," and don't wait for an offer or opportunity. You want to identify someone who takes initiative, as evidenced by actions that beat out competitors or gave the company a unique competitive advantage in response to taking action. That is, as my mentor would have said is necessary for a competitive advantage.

When interviewing top talent candidates, taking the time to understand these personality features is key to your critical analysis and final appraisal of whether they are a match. If you don't take the time to do this, and are sold on headline outcomes, you are missing a substantial amount of data that could end up costing you a lot of money when they leave prematurely.

In chapter 4, I discuss personality traits that were researched longitudinally to identify which types of traits and facets predicted professional and personal success. This study gave us a valuable tool for determining a "master checklist" for top talent that is scientific and goes beyond the "gut instinct" approach that many organizations continue to utilize.

The Organizational Self

The Organizational Self can be thought of as an avatar of the best manifestation of your Personal and Professional Self. Just like a family, an organization consists of many team members. Your Organizational Self is the extension of what you do for the organization's family members, it's mission, and to contribute to its longevity. Following the metaphor, just as there are heads of households, there are "heads of organizations," and "team leaders." In that role it is valuable to impart the best features of your Personal and Professional Self with others to help them rise to their true potential. This can be accomplished in two simple practices: Team Building & Noticing.

Team Building: There is a lot of emphasis on building strong teams. The psychology of team building actually derives from the psychology of relationships. We know from the psychology of relationships that a common need for all individuals is trust. Trust comes from the practice of non-judgement. The practice of non-judgement comes from being able to communicate in a compassionate and productive manner—the art of being a good active listener and being capable of adhering to a superordinate goal. Back in college when I was rowing in an eight-man shell, there was no "I." I counted on the other seven rowers to be pulling and focusing as hard as I was, and vice versa. This is perfect team harmony, which comes from great leadership, individual mentoring, and group coaching. With the changing workforce, and even more significant change in work-style preferences, it is even more critical to develop an organizational strategy that addresses that change. A research-driven strategy can help foster knowledge-share between older and younger team members, and leverage that knowledge through reverse-mentoring and incentives that live up to the promise of leadership development.

Noticing: When people feel noticed, they feel their efforts are appreciated. Whole campaigns are built on "appreciation marketing" for clients. Why not engage in this practice with coworkers? People can be appreciated in many ways, and to make positive habits out of this, you can make a list of your coworkers, team members, or staff and spend time thinking about their contributions and ways to meaningfully notice them.

Some possible suggestions are:

- Giving recognition in front of other team members/coworkers
- Sending them a handwritten card/note of appreciation

- Taking them out to lunch
- Providing a gift certificate to their favorite store/restaurant
- Making a donation to their favorite charity
- Offering to let them go home early on a Friday or a have a work-from-home day
- Asking them to provide a brief presentation at the next internal meeting to discuss the accomplishment and how it was done

By engaging in noticing leadership behaviors, you continue to routinely reinforce and develop positive leadership behaviors. We all have role models, and as a leader, it's your job to be the role model and nurture others' professional development to also become role models. It's a system of reciprocity. While there may be a reaction of fear that someone could take over your job if you give them all of your "tips" and "best practices," that could happen at any time by anyone. It's a wasted mental exercise. Instead, continue to focus on noticing, which naturally deposits credits in your leadership account.

CHAPTER 1 FREE BONUS DOWNLOAD:

Personal/Professional/Organizational Self-Assessment

CHAPTER 2

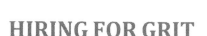

HIRING FOR GRIT

Who Are Gritty People?

In the summer of 2015, I gave a presentation on the topic of grit to a team of managers and engineers at Cisco. The presentation included a review of the psychological research on grit but also incorporated a fun exercise for everyone to rank themselves on a "grittiness" scale. The participants not only came up with keen insights about themselves, but they also reviewed the sales teams and other professionals working under them. We talked about how to further develop grit in themselves and provide feedback loops to their teams in turn to do the same. After reading this chapter, my hope is you will add this arrow to your quiver.

Dr. Angela Duckworth wrote a bestseller titled *Grit: The Power of Passion and Perseverance* and also gave a TED talk on the topic. A large body of her research looked at gritty students and how gritty kids excelled in school. She also concluded that grit could be taught to kids who were less developed in this area. Grit, as she asserts, is learnable. I agree, and the work she and another psychologist have done have made an enormous contribution to the field.

In looking at the psychological research, an abundance of studies have been conducted over the years looking at students, West Point Cadets, business professionals in the US and internationally, and college graduates who have been tracked across decades. Interestingly, most of the work prior to Duckworth didn't call those psychological features grit. There were many other personality variables, though they all relate to the same concept. In layman's language, it's called perseverance, and that research has undeniably demonstrated that many behaviors, thinking styles, and personality traits contribute to perseverance. Again, the good news is, these behaviors, thinking styles, and ways of relating with others can be identified, learned, and taught to others.

On a personal note, I have always thought about the concept of delayed gratification. In the grit research, it is often described as the capacity for engagement to long-term commitments. Delaying gratification translates to not giving up and not allowing temporary setbacks to be interpreted as failure. When I was in the midst of the arduous five years of obtaining my doctoral degree, the thought crossed my mind plenty of times. "Getting a master's degree is enough." However, I did not dwell on that thought for long. That is grit.

As an exercise, think back to some of your proudest accomplishments and reflect on the effort and time it took for those to manifest. Other than a few outlier lucky events, chances are your accomplishments came from your grittiness. If we break this down further, wherever you are at this point in time in your career, this chapter invites the opportunity to take a good look at your long-term goals and think about the long-term commitment associated to those goals.

Engaging in this thought exercise is an action we refer to in psychology as an internal locus of control. That means, you are responsible for your outcomes, your future, and the manifestation of your goals. This is contrasted by people who have an external locus of control, who expect the outside world to fulfill their needs, preferences, and goals. These folks project the absence of success onto others.

Identifying Gritty Top Talent

Many large companies have recruiters, outsourced vendors, and human resource departments with good methodology that is not always followed due to time pressure constraints. It is missing agility. The methodologies may also be limited and not tapping into the right cluster of psychological traits you are seeking. Psychological personality tests only go so far in their precision and predictability—that comment is coming from someone who has specialized in testing for almost twenty years. Smaller companies often lack the resources and human capital for comprehensive hiring. Many companies still lean heavily at the end of a hiring procedure on making hiring decisions based on "gut feelings" of candidates. So, with these limitations, let me discuss some solutions.

Another lens to look through can be borrowed from my background in forensic psychology and work in the legal system. As referred to in trial preparation, the process of hiring is a type of discovery. You are trying to discover the good and bad of your candidates. How you go about your discovery influences how informed you will be to find a gritty candidate. Trial lawyers spend countless hours on discovery preparing for a case. They believe preparation is essential, and that the most prepared win. Not a bad mindset. However, not every organization has a trial budget for hiring discovery. The good news is that technology search tools can be leveraged for efficiency to conduct discovery more efficiently and in a budget-sensitive manner.

Identifying top talent can begin with a simple grit screening questionnaire that probes candidates with various questions, tapping into grit in a non-obvious manner. It also focuses on open-ended questions, which prompt the candidate to describe in detail their past accomplishments and professional self-appraisal. Taken together, you are tapping into multiple personality traits all in one procedure, which can be handled via interview format in person, or for additional time efficiency, the candidate can be directed to complete the questionnaire online. This produces both qualitative and quantitative data to start building an internal knowledgebase for top talent hires.

At the end of this chapter is a download link for my Are You Gritty? Questionnaire that you can begin using immediately for yourself, or if you are in a position of hiring you can use it during your interview. This questionnaire helps identify, analyze, and rank the candidate's grittiness. Do they show internal locus of control thinking? Do their past achievements offer evidence of perseverance through challenge to accomplish long-term goals? Is there commensurate resilience in their personal lives? The answers to these questions will help you quickly determine whether you have a gritty candidate or not.

A fascinating 2014 study[2] looked at grit among Army Special Operations Course attendees, Chicago Public Schools high school graduates, and sales representatives of a vacation ownership company. It turns out that the people who ranked highly on grit completed the Special Operations Course, graduated high school, succeeded in their sales jobs, and when tracking men, showed that they tended to remain married. The interesting aspect of this study is the age

[2] Eskreis-Winkler Lauren, Duckworth Angela, Shulman Elizabeth, Beal Scott. (2014) The grit effect: predicting retention in the military, the workplace, school and marriage. Frontiers in Psychology, Vol. 5

differences across the developmental life span showing the robustness of the grit trait in different professional and student cohorts. Grit sticks!

Some talent and some successes can look good, sizzle, and suggest grit, but are not. It is very important to ask questions about measurable outcomes. How was success measured? How long did it take? What resources were required and what were the costs? For example, consider a candidate who reports steady sales growth under their management. Was it their management, or was their team gritty to begin with? It's important to understand the claim and the underlying data set backing the claim before making a determination.

Try to find outcomes that are directly attached to the intelligence and effort of your prospect. Results that include team effort are diluted and difficult to determine whose "talent" actually created the successful outcome. Also look at future aspirations. What personal and professional goals is your candidate setting for himself? Are they realistic? How does the candidate envision accomplishing the goals? Asking these questions will allow you to glean insights about their thinking and methodology to determine if it pairs up with past accomplishments. Successful people have a method of success that is repeatable and refinable. Finally, you want to appraise the candidate's leadership ability, which means their capacity and attitude to teach components of their method to elevate overall team performance.

When consulting with companies on both strategy and execution of hiring top talent, a structured methodology applies.

- Analysis of hiring losses of top talent in the past for better hiring precision.
- Identify company-specific human performance and character traits in existing top talent.

- Fill gaps with top talent trait assessment from the latest psychological research.

- Develop interview protocols qualitatively assessing these attributes and quantifying the results.

- Review multiple sources of data (prior co-workers, supervisors, social media) for comprehensive top talent assessment.

One of the most significant top talent hiring challenges that I believe will persist well into the next decade is the hiring of Millennials and then Generation Z workers. In addition to gauging precise top talent assessment, we know that job satisfaction is a significant influencer for retention. Having a hiring strategy that taps psychological factors associated with job satisfaction for millennials that intersects with your requirements for high performance is of great value and matters significantly in mitigating hiring losses and the costs associated with those losses.

CHAPTER 2 FREE BONUS DOWNLOAD:

Are You Gritty?

CHAPTER 3

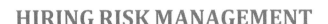

HIRING RISK MANAGEMENT

Screening for Risk Factors

In clinical psychology, we look at risk regularly. Risk of suicide, risk of violence toward others, risk of students making gun threats, and many more. We have a solid and ever-growing body of research that has evolved into a research informed model that uses various psychological instruments for assessing risk. We do this by looking at a combination of risk factors and protective factors. Risk factors are psychological liabilities, which include personality traits, thinking styles, attitudes, and of course behaviors that are destabilizing. In this model, there is no such thing as "no risk factors." Your ideal candidate would possess no elevated risk factors, meaning none are active. If you have a candidate who is a former alcoholic, that is a risk factor. If they have many years of sobriety, that risk factor is not active and is not a marker of elevated risk concern.

Protective factors are psychological assets. These include individual personality traits, healthy relationships, hobbies and interests, and other psychologically strengthening resources. Consider the alcoholic example. AA involvement would be a protective factor. So would involvement in a religious or spiritual practice, regular exercise, harmonious relationships with family and friends, and hobbies that are psychologically strengthening. Spending time getting to know your candidate in casual conversation allows for a more comprehensive understanding of these aspects to discern what risks they bring to the table and what protective factors offset those risks.

Unfortunately, most risk factors are personal, meaning that what could emerge as a problem later in the workplace is not typically driven by professional ability problems or workplace-born crises. About a year ago, I was brought in on a case involving a senior manager who had not spent much time at the company before beginning to display features of paranoia. Not much inquiry had been done on this particular hire. Ultimately, he was fired, but he continued harassing and stalking other employees at the workplace even after being fired.

If you looked at his professional qualifications on paper and in photos, you would see what appeared to be a successful, stable individual. Several weeks after the hire, when I met with this individual at his home, I was confronted with a man who had barricaded himself in his yard with a fence and set up an interrogation table with two chairs in the middle of his driveway. This was on the heels of several pending arrest warrants for violating the boundaries of former coworkers and neighbors. Even for a seasoned psychologist like me, this was a bit of an outlier.

Fortunately, we were able to navigate the man into the right mental health treatment, but this bad hire cost the company significant money in the bad hire, the replacement hire, legal fees, and the individuals whose productivity declined in response to anxiety about unpredictable retaliation until the matter was resolved with finality. The

23

dramatic point in this case example illustrates the importance of looking at personal risk factors, which often fall outside the "standard" realm of the existing hiring process.

Personal Risk Factors

Personal risk factors are frequently undetected at the time of a hire. This occurs because they are often not investigated or assessed even on a surface level of inquiry and candidate research. The four primary risk factors that have the potential to wreak significant havoc in your organization from an individual's instability come from the following list, but first a story.

A fast-growing company was seeking to replace a financial executive. It was an easy option to go with a "family friend," who appeared to have the right credentials and could easily fold right into the business. Thus, a lot of the investigative candidate research was skipped, which included checking basic credentials. The errors in this decision hinged on accepting a number of false assumptions as truth. In the end, this candidate stole a substantial sum of money from the company, destabilized the company financially, and had a major detrimental impact on the overall morale of the company leadership and capacity to remain engaged in the company mission. The latter was derailed by drawn out civil and criminal litigation that also cost significant time and legal fees. The individual was ultimately prosecuted and sentenced to federal prison on fraud. The one piece of research that would have taken about five minutes to investigate was the fact that the individual claimed to be a CPA yet possessed no registered license. His credentials fell apart from there like a house of cards.

The four primary risk factors that have the potential to wreak havoc on your organization are:

1. **Addiction**: Addiction plagues our nation, with a current epidemic of prescription opiate abuse. As I was writing this chapter someone told me about a friend who had standard hip replacement surgery (two nights in the hospital). She was sent home with seventy Percocets. Addiction can be very hard to detect, even with employee drug screens, due to the fact that there are innumerable ways to circumvent a one-time test. One way to investigate addiction is conduct a criminal background check through your state (and prior states if they have had multiple relocations) to see if there are pending charges or prior convictions associated with DWI/DUI, drug possession, etc. Any of these would be an immediate red flag that should be discussed in the interview. Conducting an internet search is also useful since it can produce police blotter results for individuals who were arrested on alcohol or drug related charges but never made it into the state criminal database because they were one-time sole offense that were triaged into a drug diversion program. If the program was successfully completed, the charge was likely removed from public record.

2. **Criminal History**: Having an arrest or criminal history is not a deal breaker, but it is definitely something to pay attention to. Criminal histories give you insights into someone's past. Was your client arrested for trespassing in college? Is there a history of domestic violence charges? Has your client ever stolen? These are risk factors to take note of in the larger picture of the behavioral analysis of your client. To identify past criminal behavior, conduct a similar research strategy as performed for addiction. Using a specific criminal background search technology, such as Intelius, can also expedite that research for a reasonable account fee that includes a national search.

3. **High Conflict Divorce**: Divorce is considered to be one of the most emotionally destabilizing life events, in the ranks of the death of a

child, death of a parent, or similar trauma. Whereas divorce is also commonplace nationally (occurring at about a 50 percent rate annually), it is something to be aware of (and inquire about during the interview.) Divorce is not so much the risk factor, but rather what is called a "high conflict divorce" (HCD). HCD occurs in about 1 percent of divorces but includes unrelenting litigation lasting years and emotional havoc and work performance disruption in response to the psychological turmoil and unending court appearances. You should ask your candidate how they are coping. How are they balancing the changes in their life? Is their time compromised by court attendance because they are in the middle of a high conflict custody battle? The answers to these questions all matter in your appraisal of having 100 percent of your client's ability, and at the very least that will help you forecast when they will be back to their full potential. You may wish to delay their onboarding if, other than the divorce, they are the best candidate.

4. **Personality Disorder**: This is probably one of the most controversial risk factors because it is perhaps impossible to detect short of your candidate announcing they have a personality problem at their interview. Personality disorders are a cluster of thinking patterns, behaviors, and emotional styles of relating with others that persistently break relationships down—your leadership, coworkers, clients. Since your candidate is unlikely to announce such problems, the strategy to detect this possibility is twofold. One is to take note of the following features during the interview:

   1. Does the candidate display all-or-nothing thinking?

   2. Does the candidate attribute all successes to oneself and all failures to others?

   3. Does the candidate disparage former leadership, company strategies, or support resources?

4. Does the candidate remark about the inadequacy of subordinates?

5. Does the candidate prefer to work in a silo away from others or alternatively control others?

6. Does the candidate remark how past performance reviews were unfair?

7. Did the candidate have at least few or no well-liked coworkers?

8. Was the candidate wildly successful but not liked by peers?

Another key strategy to investigate the risk factors of personality disorder is through reference interviews. This will give you firsthand information about others' perception of your candidates. Well-liked candidates should get glowing reviews with specific examples of positive attributes. Responses from reference interviews that are terse suggest defensiveness and a response style that is simply in service of being cooperative. Below are a number of questions that could be asked. Note that they are open-ended questions, which are designed to give you more detailed responses and the opportunity for follow-up inquiry.

- Was he/she well-liked by peers?

- How did he/she respond to feedback?

- How would you describe her/his style of relating with others?

- How would you describe his/her emotional intelligence? How would you characterize her/her leadership qualities?

In sum, everyone has risk factors, and the personal risk factors discussed in this chapter point to some of the most destructive ones a candidate may possess and bring into the company. They are not necessarily deal breakers in terms of job candidacy, but they should be scrutinized with the same degree of importance as other areas of candidate assessment.

Professional Risk Factors and Organizational Fit

This category could be thought of as reputation management. Will your candidate elevate the reputation of the company or diminish it? This matters significantly in terms of your candidate's interaction with coworkers, and secondly with customers. It's great to have passionate people, but you also want someone who can keep a lid on their personal feelings on topics that typically generate conflict-laden differences of opinion. Whereas everyone is entitled to their own beliefs and expression of belief in our country, they are not entitled to generate conflict or harassment in your workplace. This happens when people have strong beliefs, perhaps well- entrenched biases, and express those beliefs in a disrespectful and unprofessional manner. Whether or not someone does this privately on their social media accounts seen only by their followers, their public social media posts should be reviewed to learn more about your candidates and what type of communicator they are online.

CHAPTER 3 FREE BONUS DOWNLOAD:

Risk Screening Checklist

CHAPTER 4

THE BEYONDERS: A STORY OF THOSE WHO CONSISTENLY GO ABOVE AND BEYOND

The Beyonder Traits

One amazing study tracked Minnesota students for fifty years to better understand what contributed to creative achievement and personal achievement better than school grades and IQ scores. Through longitudinal tracking, the study discovered that a collection of characteristics made these successful people stand out. These are referred to as Beyond Characteristics and include the following psychological traits: love of work, high energy, persistence, sense of mission, courage, delight in deep thinking, tolerance of mistakes, feeling comfortable as a "minority of one.[3]

---

[3] Runco, M., Millar, G., Acar, S., & Cramond, B. (n.d.). Torrance Tests of Creative Thinking as Predictors of Personal and Public Achievement: A Fifty- Year Follow-Up. Creativity Research Journal, 22(4), 361–368.

One of the major contributions of this study is that it dovetails perfectly with other research on grit and positive psychology, though over a longer period, giving further validity to the factors. Let's take a moment and review these psychological traits and delve deeper into the cultivation or perhaps replenishment of them since no one can be 100 percent all of the time.

Love of Work: This equates to passion, and if you speak to anyone who truly loves what they do, they instantly convey passion. If you're unsure about your level passion, it might be time for a change. Passion is the emotional energy behind your "why" in your professional role. Take that out, and you're just a cog, right? If you've lost your passion, you should spend some time journaling what matters to you and what could reignite your energy. Maybe it's time for a change to rediscover a love of a different kind of work or a different type of role. Life is not static.

High Energy: This speaks for itself, but underlying high energy is a foundation of wellness: physical, emotional, spiritual (however you define that). If you are not physically well, it is very difficult to have consistently high energy. Psychological distress saps an enormous amount of energy. As for spirituality, psychological research has shown that people who regularly serve others are happier. So, what areas of your life can be tweaked to increase your energy? Sanjiv Chopra wrote a great short book, *The Big Five:* Five Simple Things You Can Do to Live a Longer, Healthier Life, on diet that I recommend if you're looking to make some changes there.

Mindfulness meditation can easily (and freely) help regulate your emotional and spiritual well-being. Thich Nhat Hanh wrote a short book, *Peace Is Every Step: The Path of Mindfulness in Everyday Life:* and you can download a free meditation App called Insight Timer to connect with others engaged in the same practice across the planet.

Persistence: This is grit. Never give up. The stoics (and if you're curious, you can learn a lot more at thedailystoic.com) wrote about this in the form of action taking the lead versus emotion. If you're struggling to persist, you need to understand what is detracting your attention. You need to look deeply at that and solve it. If you're struggling with persistence, you may benefit from a meeting with a trusted mentor or a coaching call consult that is personalized.

Sense of Mission: Having a sense of mission is what I like to refer to as purpose, or mattering. This attribute comes from a separation from one's ego. In terms of tangibles, this means you think about how your work matters beyond your next raise, bonus, or promotion. It refers to making a difference at a large scale of positive impact. Think SpaceX.

Courage: One can only be courageous when they have solid convictions about their own competency. If you are lacking courage, you need to identify which core and extended competencies you are lagging in and how to develop them. Doing so will give you the confidence to tolerate greater risk and do what others are unwilling to do because of fear. Fear is the antithesis of courage, and learning how to tolerate fear-management is an important skill to develop. You can try the following cognitive trick to accomplish this.

Think about your goal and what you're afraid will occur if the goal or objective is not met. Chances are, your mind has set up a number of catastrophic narratives. Now, you must acknowledge that those scripts are simply productions of the mind and not real. In reality, you can create a number of steps and actions that deliberately lead to task accomplishment. This is your fear-management pathway to build courage and overcome fear.

Delight in Deep Thinking: The creative mind is tapped into deep thinking, and this leads to innovation, invention, breakthroughs, and insights that inspire your professional development and that of your company if you are a leader. If you've never engaged in deep thinking, it can be an active or passive process. An active process of deep thinking can be journaling your thoughts on any subject. Alternatively, it can be a conversation with a friend or colleague about an abstract topic or just about anything having to do with the human experience. For me, a passive process tends to be more inspiring and comes while engaged in running or out in the mountains climbing. It tends to occur when my mind is shut off from conscious planning or thinking, and new ideas "bubble up" from my unconscious. These insights guide conscious choices that follow in personal or professional development.

Tolerance of Mistakes: The interesting point on this is that no one likes being seen as having made a mistake, but we always appreciate when someone tells us a story about a huge mistake they made. It's a classic arch of stories we all love. The challenge, the failure, the restoration, the successful ending. No one likes to focus on mistakes, but it is truly the only way to learn. Mistakes are opportunities to expedite oneself on the journey for accurate and effective solutions. To practically implement this habit requires two steps. One is to mentally accept that mistakes and errors in judgement are part of the development process. We are all fundamentally imperfect. The second is to document or mentally note when those mistakes are made never to repeat them. This may take the form of changing the way you communicate verbally or in writing or repairing a relationship. Show compassion for yourself first, and you will find it easier to demonstrate that to your coworkers and clients.

Minority of One: Being a minority of one, means being okay with having your own opinion that runs counter to group think or what everyone else in your team is thinking. Google is well-known for having a special team in which the sole purpose is to come up with moonshot ideas that on face value appear to be impossible. Your comfort level being a minority of one opens your creative self and allows for an expression of art versus logic in your quest to create practical real-world solutions to problems through innovation.

Developing Beyonders

Like any strategy, developing a team of Beyonders is no different. It requires the will to do it, defining qualities such as those outlined above, and a methodology to develop those traits in existing teams or identify and recruit new team members who already possess those traits. You will need to look at the economics of both, which is possible if you have done a quality job recruiting top talent in the first place. Your investment is best spent among the team members you already have.

Step 1: Pick one trait to work on at a time. Develop self-reporting and team response protocols to determine the one trait each person should work on for the next year. Think about the impact the trait will have individually, among the team, and globally across the organization.

Step 2: Create a buddy/partner system for accountability, and pair up partners in counterintuitive dyads to amplify the process with fresh perspectives. (male/female, creative/linear)

Step 3: Facilitate the development of daily actions to establish a habit in trait expansion. These are akin to helping a full phenotype emerge from raw genetics. If someone has the gene to be a world class swimmer, you won't see it until their practice pushes that gene for the fullest potential of its expression.

Step 4: Tie the trait to measurable outcomes and impact. This can be measured by new actions that create efficiency and effectiveness for company growth through new products, productive improvement, new services, service improvement, new clients, restored client relationships, and ultimately revenue and mitigation of losses. As a team, an additional benefit could be a greater collective consciousness, in which the synergy of everyone's actions accelerates these outcomes at a velocity that was unexpected and perhaps creates innovations that were unexpected as well.

Step 5: In the business world, getting your team together as a professional group is sometimes referred to as a "huddle" when the purpose is not solely instructive. In clinical psychology, there is a long history of group therapy, whose sole purpose is wellness development by benefitting from the group process and dynamics that would elicit key insights and feedback for its respective members. Group "process" therapy somehow got lost in the technology revolution. However, it is still a method for team-team- building and creativity that has decades of research based proven efficacy. I would like to see that value be brought back into companies as part of a top talent strategy, and for Millenials and Gen Z workers it is probably the perfect match for cultivating their strong need for 'work-life balance' and professional growth. Having someone facilitate a time-limited or ongoing "Beyonders Process Group" each week for an hour to ninety minutes can be another implementation to expand the benefits of this effort.

A Personal Story of the Benefits of Beyondering

Early in my career when I opened a forensic psychology practice, I happened to be in Boston at psychology conference and was in line at a local Starbucks. I struck up a conversation with the person behind me, who in that span of minutes scheduled a follow- up call to discuss of all things, a new software technology called Linked Entity Visualization (LEV). He was the cofounder of a start-up, based in China, that was looking for ways to visually display data sets. He immediately saw an application in forensics, as did I.

That was around 2003, and of course, we see this type of

content on TV shows, movies, etc. all of the time now. Whereas my involvement with the start-up was brief, it opened me up to a world of technology innovations that I was immediately able to apply to my business to be more efficient, effective, and agile. The point of this brief story is that it illustrates how some of my own Beyonder traits (deep thinking/curiosity) that I worked on, and I say that with full humility, helped me develop more rapidly as a professional.

CHAPTER 4 FREE BONUS DOWNLOAD:

Going Beyond Checklist

CHAPTER 5

THE EMOTIONAL INTELLIGENCE SKILLS THAT MATTER

The most successful people I know are the most emotionally intelligent. What does that mean? Emotional intelligence became popular around 1995, when psychologist Daniel Goleman wrote about it in his book, Emotional Intelligence: Why It Can Matter More Than IQ. Back in the nineties, success was heavily weighted on academics, test scores, colleges, and the like. As we now know, the world has been flipped upside down in breaking the mold of learning and career outcomes. However, we are still dreadfully lagging behind in the area of emotional intelligence. It is beyond the scope of this book to discuss the theories, yet many scientific papers have been written about it. You either accept it or you don't.

In this chapter we will focus on two specific skills associated with emotional intelligence that have been proven to have a direct impact on peak performance—communication and emotional regulation. Further, we will talk about the actions to nurture these skills, like all of the other peak performance attributes, with practice and habits designed to bring them to fruition.

First, it is necessary to point out why communication, emotional regulation, and executive functioning are not "perfect" in each of us from the start. You can easily engage in this simple exercise. Look back to your childhood and think about how good you were or were not as a speaker and listener. How was your self-control? What about delaying gratification? Self-observation? These processes start early in life, some right out of the womb, and are imprinted with environmental experiences for the better or worse that shape how we function in these domains. Neuroscience now affirms how rooted these processes become, often due to the quality of attachments with our primary caregivers. On the positive side, neuroscience also shows how changeable these processes are with proven techniques, such as mindfulness breathing or mindfulness meditation, and they can be further improved in specific types of psychotherapy.

As another exercise, I would suggest reflecting on your last project, deal, business relationship, or any other professional objective that did not come to fruition in the way you had intended. I have found in my own experience that suboptimal communication, emotional connection with others, or diminished perspective taking yielded poor results. Improving any or all of these facets of emotional intelligence can make a striking difference in performance.

Communication: Brain Based Effectiveness to Connect, Listen, and Act

We know that the most effective communication is achieved when there is active attention and listening with the other person. A helpful way to think about this is how the brain is stacked in a simple way. Layer 1 is basic needs, Layer 2 is emotional needs and Layer 3 is cognitive complexity. The following crude expression drives the point home.

You can't negotiate with a crazy person. Reasoning fails with emotionally dysregulated people. This does not mean that we're all walking around emotionally dysregulated. Yet this alerts us to the possibility that if someone is in that kind of dysregulated emotional state, and if you are unaware of it, your efforts to reason through a project, sale, proposal, etc. may be fruitless at that point in time. This communication process focuses on understanding the other person and the other person's perspective. Whether it is your team or customer, these concepts matter significantly, perhaps at all costs.

The first step to improve communication is to engage in reflective deep listening. Focus on the person and give them your full attention. Listen to what they are saying between the lines, and pay attention to their emotional state. Use reflective deep listening to show you are listening. For example, "Cathy, I'm hearing you say that this project matters a lot to you, but you're concerned we don't have the talent capacity to get it done the way you would like." Wait for the response. You will either have it correct, or it will be partially clarified. Regardless, your credibility as a good listener should increase.

When you immediately notice that something is off in an initial conversation, another way to check in is a very simple query, "Is everything okay?" If the response comes back, "Yes, why do you ask?" you can follow up with something to the effect of, "It matters to me if I can be helpful in any way beyond what we're talking about, and I just wanted to check in to let you know that." That is a non- defensive, proactive, kind response.

It can also be disarming, and you may immediately find out that someone's got a family member going through medical problems or the company is having a problem, etc. Then the new issue takes priority and that is okay. You're building trust. If it turns out that everything is okay, you've shown some vulnerability and compassion that was at the very least noticed. You put a human touch on business.

If someone is going through an emotional challenge that day (or longer), they are not likely going to be able to process the complex or perhaps even simple decision-making you might be seeking. Their brain is primarily thinking about the emotional issue and trying to resolve that challenge. That's what matters most to that person at that moment. If you are trusted, you may be invited to help. If you are in new relationship, you won't be, but you can propose having a follow-up conversation at a different time. Try to identify (or ask) for a follow-up when matters are better. Depending on circumstances, that could be a day, a week, a month, or longer.

In the process of deep listening, you can also show emotional appreciation to the other person about what you admire in them. Let me be clear. This is not to be patronizing and is based on the assumption that you are truly invested in your team or customer. For example, "Cathy I know you are recognized in your company as a leader, and you're extremely well-liked by many people we both work with. I really appreciate what you've done professionally and it matters to me that our collaboration only enhances that."

Proposals as Preferences

We make proposals all day long to ourselves and others. What should I eat for breakfast? What will I tackle first today? When it comes to effective communication, we hit a wall when our proposals are rejected or are met with an unseen obstacle. The way around this is not to take it personally, but instead to ask permission to make a counter proposal, or several proposal variations. The same methodology applies to work in teams, assignment of projects, sales, and just about anything else.

Rejection of a proposal often triggers a fight or flight response. This equates to an emotional reaction and further pushing of your preferences, or withdrawal and acceptance of defeat. The alternative is again to respond with "Would it make a difference if…?" or "Can I have the opportunity to modify the proposal, give you a different solution, come up with a different strategy?" Then you have to find out what was misaligned with the original proposal and propose a new and better solution. How do you figure it out? Ask! What didn't fit with what I proposed? How would you prefer this project gets underway? Includes? Is approached? Issue resolved? The proposal and counterproposal process, when done effectively, can go back and forth many times, as long as there is ongoing clarification of what the other person is seeking. That is the key. Figure it out, and then offer it.

Emotional Regulation

We all have demands placed on us each day that pose the challenge to either react, or the opportunity to pause, observe, and take deliberate action. The latter requires emotional regulation, the ability to "cool your jets" and be aware of the emotional pushes and pulls behind the demands, and ultimately the people putting them on us. This can come in the form of a project delayed, errors, team conflict, or unrealistic expectations placed on us.

First it is helpful to understand where the cornerstones of emotional regulation come from. This is a neurological phenomenon and psychological process we have all been exposed to since birth. It comes from the attachment process between the infant and the primary caregiver. Is the infant reassured that the world is a safe place, and when posed with conflict, is the infant reassured by the caregiver? Or is the world frightening and there is an absence of consistent reassurance. These psychobiological mechanisms prime the emotional regulation system in the body that establishes the framework for how we relate with others as we go through life.

For those fortunate enough to have had healthy attachments, they go on to relate well with others, show compassion, and don't generally get pulled into emotional conflict. For those who were less fortunate, a fight or flight response can be triggered, followed by actions in either of those directions. Conflict avoidance or conflict seeking, in short. For others, emotional regulation and repairing it is their own psychological work. If you find yourself needing a tune- up in this area, you can do the work and get good outcomes.

Again, without going too deep into the science, we're talking about developing a technique to teach the body and mind how to calm itself. Since we are biologically based, the techniques are quite natural and begin with simple breathing. Breathing exercises, in just a few minutes, have been proven to alter one's brain state by regulating blood pressure, pulse rate, and tension. This happens naturally by slowing your breathing and simply noticing your breathing. Breathe in, Breathe out. Do this ten times, and you will notice a difference. Stay with it for as long as you need, though most find that they are back to a calmer state in less than five minutes and able to reason with better clarity by departing from an emotional reaction.

There are many variations of this, and it is formally taught through a technique called Mindfulness Meditation. There as many types of mindfulness meditation as there are stars in the galaxy, but it need not go any further than breathing. A nifty app, and one that I personally use, is called Insight Timer and is mentioned several times in this book. No, I don't get any financial benefit for recommending it, I simply believe it is very good, and it's free. You have the option to breathe (meditate) in silence or with any one of thousands of guided meditations for as short or long as you like.

I have found that beginning the day with mindful meditation is great way to clear the mind, be open to opportunity, and to simply let your positive self emerge for the day. Following the same technique any time during the day has equal benefit but can serve as a great tool for practice with no training and no materials, anywhere at all.

In the midst of conflict, being able to stay emotionally regulated gives you the advantage of observing the conflict versus being drawn into it through reaction. It is a way to take peaceful action. With all of the technology advances, we can expect new devices, particularly through Virtual Reality and Augmented Reality, to provide additional tools for regulation and entering our "flow state" to create more fluid work environments both individually and for teams. Stay in touch with me if those are the kinds of workshop experiences you are interested in having!

CHAPTER 5 FREE BONUS DOWNLOAD:

The 1 Minute Method To Make Better Decisions

CHAPTER 6

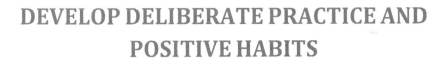

DEVELOP DELIBERATE PRACTICE AND POSITIVE HABITS

Why Deliberate Practice Matters

Have you ever started out with the intention of establishing a new positive habit... and Failed? You're not alone.

A longitudinal study in the *Journal of Behavioral Medicine* showed that about 50 percent of new gym members quit before the six-week mark. Why would people who want to look good, feel healthy, or lose weight just quit?

I will explain the simple principles of what habit research shows, but most importantly, I will teach you in a two minute solution to develop and sustain high performance habits.

The gym member study I just mentioned is consistent with plenty of other habit research. The answer is not intention. It matters less what you intend to do. Everyone has good intentions in the beginning and even on an ongoing basis.

The answer is also not mood, or being positive. Mood changes. Just look at your last twenty-four hours. Mine had distractions just like yours.

What's the solution? Consistency.

This comes as no surprise in the realm of high performance behavior research. The term "Deliberate Practice" has been associated with elite performance by top performers, and even children in The Growth Mindset research by Carol Dweck. This will be discussed in greater depth in chapter 9. For now, just recognize that deliberate practice is the first step in establishing a routine of positive habit creation. This is a proven method to get the outcomes you are seeking.

All top performers have mastered this: The Rolling Stones, Michael Phelps, and you. A similar angle on this was written in Malcolm Gladwell's bestseller, *Outliers* where a research study demonstrating that mastery comes after ten thousand hours of practice was expanded upon. Think of it this way. Ten thousand hours of practice need not be literal, but rather thought of more collectively in terms of reading, writing, and a wealth of life experiences aimed at a common objective. You're probably closer to 10,000 hours than you thought.

A Case Study

A sales executive wanted to increase referrals from existing clients.

Here's how the habit was developed:

1. **Goal:** Deepen engagement with customers for new sales from their lead network.
2. **Habit:** Spend time learning more about the customers' interests and needs to give added value.
3. **Deliberate Practice Sessions:** Research the customer deeper. Have conversations with the customer without any intention of selling. Going "three layers deep" to understand the customers' deepest problems. Then give generous solutions derived from these conversations.
4. **Outcome:** Ask the customer for new lead introductions after delivering valuable insights.

Scheduling Habits and Follow-Through

Scheduling may be one of the easiest but most elusive obstacles for positive habit creation and follow-through. More than ever, we have structured schedules on our smart phone with reminders. Short of mistyping a date or time, it's almost impossible to miss a meeting. The people I know who are consistently late either don't use a schedule, a reminder, or both. Scheduling is one of the best ways to make sure new habits take hold. If it's in your calendar, it's a lot more difficult to blow off a task you're trying to implement that is a stepping stone to a new objective. People who do not schedule these tasks are less likely to implement them. Scheduling tasks associated with your positive habit creates the "stickiness" of follow-through.

Three Tips You Can Immediately Use

Identify your goal with great specificity. This could be creating more sales interactions, improving relationships with clients by giving high-value information, developing a proposal for a strategy or product, publishing an article, etc.

Schedule a consistent time of day you will engage in your practice, put it on your calendar, and never break it.

Beyond the six weeks, you need to maintain your habit with the principle of consistency. Engage in the task or effort at the same time every day. This creates the "stickiness" of habit.

Another tactical action you can take is to pair up with a co-worker who is also committed to improvement and deliberately work on one aspect of professional development. Schedule a time to talk or meet in person at a frequency you both prefer. At least once weekly is recommended in person, but touching base remotely as often as is supportive for both of you is even more beneficial.

Leveraging Technology for Habit Making

Depending on your objective, there may be ways to leverage technology for a small investment that can give you high returns, over a shorter period of time. For example, initiatives associated with sales and marketing require customer research and other market data analysis. You can outsource a lot of this research with a virtual research assistant who is a graduate student either in the US or another country as long as they have access to research material references that are commensurate with your needs. In my own discipline I have used graduate students locally, but also in other countries who are English speaking.

Another common objective may pertain to the presentation of data or other types of presentations. Once the research is done, you can outsource the actual development of slides regardless of the application you use. Using high quality visual images from photo databases can also make a high impact.

Almost everyone uses a CRM platform. Adding customer information can be time consuming and detract your attention from more important objectives. Nonetheless, having comprehensive data allows you to strengthen relationships over time. Outsourcing data entry into your CRM can also be done quite easily. For example, dictate the information you want added, and email, or Dropbox the file to your transcriptionist or data entry assistant. You can accomplish the dictation while commuting to save additional time.

Keeping the Positive Habits Flowing

Deliberate practice in the service of positive habit making is a central tenet of top performers. They are always polishing good habits and creating new ones through the same methodology. Once you improve the skill you are working on, there will always be a next one as long as you are committed to this level of professionalism and expertise. Having a professional colleague or small group of like- minded professionals can be beneficial in helping you stay on point. Everyone hits walls in this process, and having objective feedback through professional development coaching can be an asset to help reveal an unseen weakness and draw out an untapped or underutilized talent. Coaching can help formulate a missing component of a strategy to help you accomplish your goals quicker.

CHAPTER 6 FREE BONUS DOWNLOAD:

Your Positive Habit Strategy & Schedule

CHAPTER 7

BUILD DEEP CUSTOMER APPRECIATION

What Is Deep Customer Appreciation?

The best companies are experts in providing customized appreciation to their buyers or customers. If you accept the definition that the sole purpose of any business is to generate a profit, this model consists of a financial transaction between a buyer and seller. The buyer trusts the seller is providing the value in the product or service to meet their expectations. The best companies exceed those expectations.

In general, at the beginning of most sales, there is no de-facto expectation by the customer that they will be appreciated, liked, or treated in a way that goes beyond courtesy. With this backdrop, we now see a lot of "rewards programs," which are designed to reward the customer for repeated purchases. The limitation of this model is that it is tied to the financial transaction. If you buy more x, we will give you y. Technology has come so far that it can now track our purchases and position future products and services in front of us that we are more likely to buy again or try. This is clever marketing, but not true customer appreciation.

True customer appreciation is earned. It is earned by spending time and effort to get to know the person, and what matters to them in the deepest way possible. To think of it differently, have you ever considered buying something, or actually did so, after a close friend recommended it? Why did you do that? Beyond the surface issues, it was likely because you trust them and that they know what you like and what matters most to you. You trust that they care about you, the person, and less so whether you actually buy the product or service being discussed. This same approach should be taken with true customers.

The first step is to learn to develop an appreciation for their interests, needs, and preferences professionally. The second step is to learn the same about them personally. The method to implement this approach requires spending time just "hanging out" and getting to know your customer better. Traditionally, this happens over coffees or meals. I would propose that spending time at other social and recreational functions poses equal if not better advantages. For example, you could invite your customer as a guest to a fundraiser. These are typically social events (wine tastings, art exhibits, fundraising road races, etc.) that are low pressure environments for high quality conversation. If you are invited to those types of events, you should go. Again, it will give you deeper insights about what matters most to your customer and help you develop solutions that are properly aligned with their professional and personal interests.

Identifying Customer Wants and Needs

Getting to know your customer is like any courtship. Beyond the transaction of the sale and aligning the needs and goals of that transaction, the work is to develop a relationship that supports trust.

Trust is the belief that the person behind the transaction will complete it as requested. Remember, past transactions have failed. Promises have been broken. To accomplish this, you are acknowledging that the customer has a number of fears about why the deal/project/outcome could fail in any way.

You must instill confidence in your customer that you will not allow this failure. Your work is therefore to uncover the fears. After calls and meetings, you should make a simple list of these fears by paying close attention to what is said during those conversations. Is there a fear of under budgeting? Not meeting deadlines? The product or service may not do what is promised? Figure out these fears and develop answers (solutions) to overcome those fears with great authority and confidence.

This will show that you are listening and not simply selling. One approach that works in all relationships is the notion of asking permission. If you ask permission, you instantly create a preliminary space for trustful conversation. After all, the person has the option to say no. You are asking and practically guaranteed to get a yes. You can do this in any manner that feels comfortable to you and is contextually relevant. Here are some examples where I use the word "project," which could be replaced with any condition of your interaction:

- Can I ask what is most important about this project?
- Can you explain what matters most about this project?
- Can you give me an example of what has gone wrong on prior projects?
- Can you help me understand the most critical components for the outcome you are seeking?
- Is there any feedback or concerns you have with my proposal that I can address?

Once you have this feedback, continue to probe deeper. Show validation. (I appreciate that feedback. I appreciate you telling me that. I understand how that can be an issue.)

This can be followed by a request. Can I have the opportunity to address these concerns/issues and show you how I will make this the right solution? Your desire to refine your proposal is born out of your refining process of understanding your client. For example, when one customer came to me asking for a hiring solution. Embedded in their fear was not having ample staff in their business to utilize the information I was providing. So what did I do? I couldn't put staff in their business as a solution. So, I asked questions to understand what that missing staff would theoretically do, and then I added that work to the proposal. I added more value at no additional cost. In that example, the solution became twofold. One solution was providing a hiring methodology to mitigate risks and maximize talent recruitment, but the other was to do it in a way that fit into their existing understaffed hiring workflow.

These instances of transaction are free opportunities to get to know your customer personally and equally understand what matters to them. What are they working on in terms of their professional development? What curiosities or interests do they have? What hobbies are fulfilling to them? By uncovering this information, you can become a temporary ambassador to their professional and personal goals. You might introduce them to someone who can help them further. You may be aware of an expert in one of those areas. You may have any number of resources (or be able to uncover them) and freely give them to your client.

This goes back to the "mattering" concept but emerges through permission-based questions and building trust. This creates an opportunity to build a business friendship, and when you add this person to your CRM system, you now have a comprehensive dossier of these important attributes. You should set reminders, in an appropriate way, to continue to provide high-value resources (information, introductions, etc.) to this person, and you will have proven you are a high quality professional.

Case Study: In another meeting when planning a presentation, I had a customer disclose to me that they were struggling with depression in spite of having a highly successful career. This was an easy solution for me. The challenge was she worked an excessive number of hours and traveled a lot. I figured out where it would be most practically convenient for her to have a therapy session in person and also suggested some might be virtual. Then I gave him the name of someone I knew who was both competent and capable of matching her work schedule. I made the appropriate introductions the same day in a matter of hours. Instant solution and infinite trust.

Developing deep appreciation places an emphasis on getting to know your customers at a level deeper than is typical. By following the steps and types of questions described, you can do this very simply. A good friend of mine gave me a tip on this years ago that is so simple it's shocking. He simply asks, "What do you do for fun?" It's a very simple, noninvasive, but highly revealing question. You will instantly know something important about your client. You need to be ready to answer the same question. Be honest and share something about yourself that they may not expect. This will deepen conversation naturally in a way that creates vulnerability. This vulnerability is good, meaning a level of trust is being cultivated.

CHAPTER 7 FREE BONUS DOWNLOAD:

How To Instantly Relax An Agitated Customer

CHAPTER 8

RETAIN: THE GROWTH MINDSET

Why Lifelong Learning Matters

Psychologist Carol Dweck brought the concept of the Growth Mindset to the forefront of attention regarding its relevance to high performers and as a proven method to continually up one's game and have a competitive advantage. The advantage in this regard is committing oneself to "bettering" through consistent action aimed at learning and applying that knowledge.

With so many sources of information available at our fingertips, it is far easier than in decades past to leverage knowledge, which anecdotally, was written about when technology tools first emerged as sources of knowledge management. Who would have imagined how many options would exist today that leverage efficiency. Simple examples are podcasts, TED talks, and audio books that can be used during any commute. They can also be used during breaks, working lunches, and evening hours. Best of all, many of these knowledge resources are free or of minimal cost when compared to the price of going to business conferences and the lost work time.

The Growth Mindset also nicely dovetails with the 80/20 rule, giving us the ability to focus and maximize 20 percent of effort toward our most important objectives. Here's a real world example. If your objective is to learn any new skill or strategy and your average daily commute is sixty minutes round trip, you can now use 5 hours every week to complete a series of podcasts, TED talks, or an audiobook. Subtracting a month of a vacation time, that opens up the opportunity for 240 new learning hours aimed at high performance objectives!

5 hours/week=240 hours annually

240 hours annually=240 new insights, skills, and strategies annually

When you add this up over time, you see how when setting long-term goals, you can expedite and optimize your own learning curve to accomplish that task. Yes, this may come with the sacrifice of not listening to your favorite music or catching up on the latest series of Netflix, but if you're in the business of high performance, you will be the expert behind the content of the "next best" in your industry. Would you rather be the performer or the viewer? Paying or being paid for your high value? Conceptually, it's as simple as that. In Chapter 6, we discussed the importance of the practice of scheduling and positive habits. This is the precise concrete methodology to accomplish this.

The reality is no one is perfect. We all have highs and lows, and we all get stuck at times in the push-pull tension between motivation and action.

It's human nature, and some of us are better at this than others. I have found that having a philosophy as an underlying storyline that stands the test of time has been helpful as a daily reminder.

Some people read religious teachings, engage in spiritual practice, meditate, etc. As discussed in Chapter 5, the practice of mindfulness is one I could subjectively discuss both from a scientific standpoint and from my own practice, for its positive impact on hitting the reset button each morning to disconnect from the mind, open awareness, and reflect on the "why" of what I am doing. This creates the opportunity for results I am seeking in a state of relaxation and on really good days free of mental distraction.

Following my meditation each morning, I receive a short writing from The Daily Stoic which is the philosophy I have currently chosen to adopt that focuses on action, not emotion, and definitely not motivation. I prefer this philosophy because emotions and emotional states are, from a psychological standpoint, what we call dynamic. They constantly change. If I was only taking deliberate action when I felt great, that would significantly diminish my effective and efficient productivity. Same for motivation. Our bodies and mental states go through cycles. Committing to action eradicates those rationalizations and realities of the human condition. By taking action, and committing to it on a daily basis, we can easily adopt the Growth Mindset and the actions that are part and parcel of this way of life.

Another aspect of the Growth Mindset that I have found beneficial is what I will call experimental creative learning. For myself as a psychologist, I was immersing myself, putting attention, effort, and time into learning about emerging technologies and their applications. Each year for several years I attended the MIT CIO symposium in Cambridge, where radical technologies pertaining to cloud-computing, robotics, artificial intelligence, and many profound breakthroughs were being taught.

The vendors at these conferences were breakthrough technology companies with technology so new sometimes the service or product wasn't even available yet, but I was the first to see the "Coming Soon" attractions. There were also book vendors with the latest (as far as print goes) writings on these inventors and scientists. I had no tangible application to immediately use the knowledge in this venue, but each year it opened my mind and helped me build various applications into my brick and mortar practice and digital business services. This type of immersion can take many forms, and exploring those forums is encouraged. It could be art, history, poetry, astronomy, or even something physical. The point is to open up an area of the brain that is not routinely active.

Promoting the Growth Mindset with Precision

The human brain thrives on novelty. In the most simplistic example, Dopamine, the neurotransmitter responsible for pleasurable feelings, increases during novel experiences. The relevance to the Growth Mindset is to throw all kinds of curve balls at the brain. Read, listen, watch, interact and engage. We all have various sensory preferences for learning — auditory, visual, kinesthetic, verbal — though we can still learn through our less preferred senses. As an accompaniment to the practice of Growth Mindset learning activities, sometimes I highlight, take notes, reflect and later write in my journal or create a follow-up "to-do reading list" to read an original or supplementary source of content. By example, this book is chock full of them.

It's helpful to know your preferred learning sensory style and make sure you're loading up your knowledge content in that medium as much as possible. Be sure to build a library over time. If you're an author on any social media platform, internally or publicly, this is your opportunity to teach what you learn, share your knowledge, and connect with like-minded learners. In truth, you're positioning yourself with action steps to constantly improve your learning while also gaining recognition as a thought leader on authoritative subject matter.

Case Study: In a recent meeting with a friend who is a computer engineer for Google, he shared how he spends his commute watching YouTube Videos followed by an onsite gym workout. If you were thinking the YouTube videos were the latest comedy specials, you were wrong. The videos were a variety of knowledge trainings on many different subjects. This is how high performers take action with the Growth Mindset.

CHAPTER 8 FREE BONUS DOWNLOAD:

Becoming An Expert With Growth Mindset Strategies

CHAPTER 9

RETAIN: MENTORING AND COACHING

All successful people have at some point in their lives had a mentor. Many successful people sustain ongoing relationships with their coaches and mentors, and enjoy the benefit of having objective strategic feedback in a trusted relationship. This may take the form of weekly videoconference meetings followed by biweekly meetings, quarterly, biannually or something completely hybrid. It all depends on your needs.

Prior to identifying the right coach, it is important to identify your personal goals and dreams. This is your "why." By doing this, you tap into the emotional part of your brain that has a lot of influence on your daily state. Even though we talked about not relying on motivation, but instead action, to achieve your goals, it's still important to know why you are working so hard to succeed in the first place. This can be a fun and easy activity, only requiring your purchase of a journal (or a piece of paper) to write down your personal and professional goals. This should be a brainstorming activity in which you don't judge any of your ideas. When you give yourself the space and time to reflect on "what matters," you may be surprised what rises to the surface and lands on paper.

Here's one example of personal and professional goals:

Personal Goals:

1. Earn more money to take the family on an extended trip outside the US each year.
2. Learn to ski.
3. Have time to learn to play guitar.

Professional Goals:

1. Become a manager/vice-president in my current organization.
2. Position myself for a better job with company that I've always wanted to work for.
3. Earn enough skills to work on a side-project and maybe position myself to be an entrepreneur.

Once you develop your lists, you can share them with your mentor. This will help your mentor truly understand what you are seeking to accomplish, and from there fine tune a granular strategy. If you opt to write down these goals in your journal, you have the advantage of looking back over time and seeing how many you've accomplished, or alternatively, how the goals may change with different life experiences.

How Do I Find a Mentor?

There are many ways to find a mentor, but the simplest way I have found is by contacting friends and family. Why? You have already established trust in this circle, and getting an introduction to a potential mentor will be far easier than if you are a stranger. Prior to reaching out to friends and family, you should determine what type of mentoring you are seeking. Spend sufficient time on this and be specific. Identify whether you are seeking mentoring to learn a new skill or set of knowledge, or you are seeking strategic mentorship. Here's a few examples.

Learning a new skill:

- I want to learn how to be a better writer in professional publications.
- I am seeking to be better at motivating and giving feedback to my team.
- I want to get feedback on how I can make my time more efficient and productive each day.

Learning a strategy:

- I'm very good at what I do, but I'm not being recognized as a leader.
- I need to perform better than my competition in a specific area, but I'm not sure how to start.
- I want to learn how to test a business idea for a product or service.

Once you've identified what you are seeking, you are ready to communicate your intention to your friends and family through email or phone calls. Keep this very personal since it is your closest circle. An example of an email is as follows:

Dear Uncle Joe,

Warm greetings from Chicago! I hope you and Aunt Jane are enjoying your summer. My career has been terrific so far, and I'm working on improving my role in the company. To that point, I am currently looking for a mentor to help me develop some leadership skills. Is there someone you could introduce me to who may be able to help me with this type of mentoring? I appreciate your assistance and input. If you'd like to discuss it over a call, just let me know.

With the type of email above, you are instantly tapping into a larger network. Even if you don't have family who are useful in this type of networking, reach out to your friends. One of my close friend's father was a retired executive who was extremely successful. I had not seen or spoken to him in a few decades, but after being re-introduced he was delighted to help me work on a specific strategy at the time. This was accomplished over virtual meetings on an as-needed basis.

How to Benefit the Most from Being Mentored

There's a few useful maxims to make a mentoring relationship successful for both you and your mentor. If done properly it can yield many years of tremendous advantage for you and be personally rewarding for them.

- Always write your questions in advance, think them through, edit and then send them ideally on one short page.
- Be prepared and punctual for your meetings. Be ready to take notes, and think about follow-up questions that have emerged since you wrote your first list of questions. If agreeable, record the calls so you can listen back.
- Be sure you understand the feedback you are getting and how to use that feedback to set milestones for your desired objective. If it's not clear, get clarification.
- Set up parameters for your next meeting, either on a specific time, typically driven by a specific milestone accomplishment, when you'll need your next step of feedback.

Daily Strategy Sheets

When working on high performance skills, it can be helpful to use a daily strategy sheet [https://hiringtoptalent.com/top-talent-book-bonus-sign-up/] when you're first establishing these habits and scheduling your time. As you can see on the sheet, you list your daily goal on the top, the milestones underneath, and the daily actions to accomplish the daily goals. From there, you schedule the time to match your actions. This is truly a foolproof system, and it feels good at the end of the day, or during your day, to check off your accomplishments of those actions, and ultimately your daily goal. This takes less than five minutes and you should do it first thing in the morning.

Agile Coaching

Coaching is different than mentoring in a number of ways, particularly in that it adds a degree of personalization to the relationship that mentoring typically does not. As described, mentoring is very issue focused. Coaching can be that, but it is often much more. It brings the unique value of the coach's education, knowledge, and experience into the dialogues.

As a psychologist who specialized in assessment for twenty years, I offer a unique advantage to quickly listen and precisely pinpoint the intersection between personal and professional needs. For example, one client started a conversation telling me he was feeling "burnt out," which led to the revelation that there was a lot of pressure on the professional side to increase sales volumes. But on the personal side, he was dealing with depression and guilt over being away from family so much. We tackled both fronts.

The agile coaching I recommend spans six weeks and is oriented around this time frame for positive habit development that immediately impacts high performance success. Agile coaching includes video phone conferencing or in-person meetings and follow-up communication via email. Your coaching plan should include an initial assessment and then feedback about your relative strengths and weaknesses, a strategic plan that responds to your MDO (Most Desired Objective), resources and practices to create the action behind your objective, and consistent sessions during the six weeks with your coach for accountability.

CHAPTER 10

A RENEWABLE FLOW STATE:
365 DAYS OF HIGH PERFORMANCE

The mind-body connection has been scientifically proven with studies showing the benefits of nutritious foods, sleep, meditation, exercise, connections with partners and friends, and play (vacation). A relevant quote from the recent movie *Christopher Robin*, has Winnie the Pooh reminding Christopher, who at this point in time in the movie is a high performer executive for the Winslow Luggage Company, that, "Nothing always leads to something." This was the paradoxical message about always grinding away versus having time for friends and play. Why do you think Google buildings have a room with Legos in them and Scooters for getting down the hallway?

There are several key methods and principles to maintain High Performance. No one is perfect, and no one is "on" daily. We all go through cycles of physical strength, wellness, and creativity, but we also fatigue in all of those respective domains. It is important to replenish oneself and in those down phases take the time to allow inspiration to emerge, the body to rest, and the mind to be less constrained. These are great times to indulge in things like a massage for the body, a mini vacation/retreat, a new exercise you've never tried, or maybe some quality time with friends and family you have not seen recently.

Aside from those down days in your cycle, having someone to connect with, like a "buddy system" on a weekly or monthly basis, can assist you with accountability. Many high performers will say they are self-driven and don't need that connection, but I believe having someone who is supportive and adds to your accountability also helps you reach your potential more regularly. Your 'buddy' can simply be someone who is working on professional improvement in an area of their life. They do not need to be related to you. This could be an exercise partner, someone you have lunch with routinely who eats healthy, or a coworker who you share apps or Growth Mindset learnings with. Rotate your buddy system around, make new connections, and be helpful to others, and you will be on the right path.

Weekly Positive Habits / Novelty Matters

Every week you should keep track of your basic needs to reach your top potential. You can take note of this formally on a worksheet like the one listed below and switch it up each month, or you can modify it on a weekly basis.

Again, novelty matters, so switch it up weekly, biweekly, or monthly to keep your growth dynamic and challenging.

High Performance Habit Domains	WEEKLY HABITS
Nutrition	Add in healthy snacks (nuts and protein bar)
Exercise	Start new strength training. Yoga 1x weekly
Learning	New TED podcast links set in browser
Clients	Deep research on one client daily and connect
Leadership	Research daily for thirty min, and write one article on LinkedIn.

Personalized Cycles of Performance: Preventing Burnout by Pivoting

Superordinate Goals

To truly maximize the benefits of positive psychology and high performance, goal setting is important. It's always easy to set goals that you can ultimately accomplish. The real challenge comes from setting goals for the seemingly impossible. Peter Diamandis is famous for his X

Prize competition each year, which awards exactly that type of outcome. If we don't challenge the impossible, we limit our growth.

It's important to realize that beyond a base layer of professional goals, high performers tend to have superordinate goals. These goals are more far-reaching than a paycheck or promotion. They are innovative, change-making, and often have outcomes that positively impact others in a way that matters to a broader community. Spend some time thinking about your superordinate goals.

Regardless, it is also okay if you are not at a place in your life where you have a superordinate goal in mind. Be open to that opportunity and how you may empower it once you have discovered it. This could turn out to be your "super power" that propels your professional development ahead at great velocity.

Retreats and Replenishing

In my profession as a psychologist, we call taking a day off to decompress a "mental health day." The benefit holds true for any professional. In the work of high performance, it is important to replenish regularly. This may mean taking a morning or afternoon off, a full day, and long weekends on a quarterly or tri-annual basis to have rest, but it can also mean you reflect and focus on your accomplishments and future directions.

I have the good fortune of having a wellness center in my building that offers yoga, massage, and has salt water float tanks. This is an easy way for a spontaneous decompression followed by reflective writing afterward. For me, extended replenishment comes through mountain climbing, usually in the Colorado Rocky Mountains. The high altitude slow steady pace going uphill becomes a liberating meditation in the wild and rugged outdoor elements. I find myself coming back replenished, in spite of the physical labor, and with new insights having given my mind a break from the typical routines and decisions and instead being attentive to safety, the weather, and precise movements of hands and feet on mountain peaks. Find your own places near or far, and ideally where you can both replenish and create a renewable flow state of top performance.

Epilogue: Take Action!

I hope you enjoyed this book and have discovered new insights for yourself, your team, or your organization.

Take action! If you follow the guiding points in this book, you will succeed and achieve your goals. Sometimes taking the first step is the hardest. If you found this book beneficial, I invite you to stay connected with me on my private top talent membership list. You will receive the latest applicable psychological research on high performance, webinar invitations, and discounts on coaching and other services I offer. I never share any of your personal information!

Stay connected with me and the Top Talent Community!

www.toptalentpsychology.com

Lastly, if you found this book beneficial, please share it and spread the optimism. Let people know, write a book review, or invite me to come speak at your company.

FREE BOOK BONUS DOWNLOADS ARE HERE:

https://hiringtoptalent.com/top-talent-book-bonus-sign-up/

Made in the USA
Middletown, DE
30 July 2021

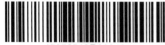

45053518R00043